THIS PLANNER

Belongs To:

Ashlee + Marli ♡

I'm PREGNANT!

How I found out

My reaction

At home pregnancy test. TOOK 2. Then went to clinic and confirmed I was shocked. I couldn't believe it. I was very happy though.

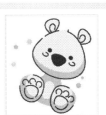

WHAT I AM MOST EXCITED ABOUT

I am most excited about teaching and learning with my baby. I'm also excited to see Isaac be a dad. I am also excited about my mom being an involved grandma.

WHO I TOLD FIRST

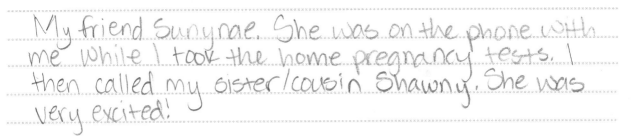

My friend Sunynae. She was on the phone with me while I took the home pregnancy tests. I then called my sister/cousin Shawny. She was very excited!

WHAT I WANT YOU TO KNOW

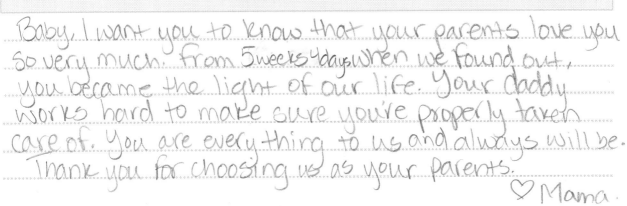

Baby, I want you to know that your parents love you so very much. From 5 weeks 4 days when we found out, you became the light of our life. Your daddy works hard to make sure you're properly taken care of. You are everything to us and always will be. Thank you for choosing us as your parents.

♡ Mama.

MY BIRTH PLAN *Ideas*

♥♥♥♥♥♥♥♥♥♥♥♥♥♥♥♥♥♥♥♥♥♥♥♥♥♥♥♥♥♥♥♥♥

WHO I WANT IN THE DELIVERY ROOM:

TYPE OF BIRTH

- [ ] **VAGINAL**
- [ ] **WATER BIRTH**
- [ ] **C-SECTION**
- [ ] **VBAC**

THOUGHTS ABOUT BIRTH AND WHAT IS MOST IMPORTANT TO ME

GETTING READY FOR THE BIG DAY: TO DO

NOTES & IDEAS (lighting, music, etc.)

40 Weeks

PREGNANCY *Tracker*

Keep track of how you're feeling every week of your pregnancy.

1	2	3	4	5	6	7
8	9	10	11	12	13	14
15	16	17	18	19	20	21
22	23	24	25	26	27	28
29	30	31	32	33	34	35
36	37	38	39	40		

APPOINTMENT *Tracker*

♥♥♥♥♥♥♥♥♥♥♥♥♥♥♥♥♥♥♥

Keep track of your pre-natal classes and doctor appointments.

DATE	TIME	ADDRESS	PURPOSE
11/2/21	2:00pm	5900 Hillandale Lithonia, GA	1st appointment
11/9/21	2:45pm	''	1st ultrasound

BABY SHOPPING *List*

Start planning for the arrival of your baby by using the shopping list below.

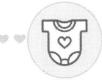

Undershirts	Crib	Bottles
Socks	Bassinet	Bottle Liners
Pajamas	Baby Bath tub	Nursing Bra & Pads
Sweaters	Car Seat	Breast Pump
Onesies	Stroller	Formula
Hats	High Chair	Pacifiers
Bibs	Play Pen	Bottle Brush
Blanket	Baby Swing	Burp Cloths
Diaper Bag	Monitor	Bottle Sanitizer
Mitts	Change Table	Nipples
Diapers	Rocking Chair	Baby Powder
Booties	Night Light	Baby Wipes
Receiving Blankets	Mobile	
Crib Sheet	Bouncer	
Wash Cloths	Nail Clippers	
Towels	Teething Toys	
	Baby Wipes	
	Diaper Pail	

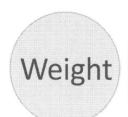

Weight PREGNANCY Tracker

 Weight Tracker Chart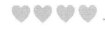

It's important to keep track of your weight throughout your pregnancy.
Record your weight in the chart below every week, starting at week 4.

WEEKLY WEIGHT TRACKER

Week	Weight	Week	Weight	Week	Weight	Week	Weight	Week	Weight
4		12		20		28		36	
5		13		21		29		37	
6	160	14		22		30		38	
7		15		23		31		39	
8		16		24		32		40	
9		17		25		33			
10		18		26		34			
11		19		27		35			

NOTE

According to the American Pregnancy Association, pregnant women should consume up to 300 more calories a day. Further, healthy eating is critical to your baby's development which means you should make sure to maintain a well-balanced diet, high in nutrients and proteins.

HEALTHY FOOD Ideas

VEGETABLES & LOW SUGAR FRUIT	PROTEINS	COMPLEX CARBS	HEALTHY FATS	SUPPLEMENTS
Leafy greens (spinach, etc.)	Organic meat	Beets	Avocado	Vitamin D
Broccoli	Liver	Carrots	Olive Oil	Fish Oil
Cauliflower	Bone Broth	Sweet Potatoes	Coconut Oil	Algae Oil
Cabbage	Beans	Yams	Yogurt	Probiotics
Asparagus	Lentils	Parsnips	Almonds	Ginger Pills
Cucumber	Flax Seed	Turnips	Mixed Nuts	Licorice Root
Mushrooms	Pumpkin Seed	Pumpkin	Soybean	Magnesium
Celery	Chia Seed	Buckwheat	Olives	Krill Oil
Radish	Salmon	Brown Rice	Nut butter	Iron Pills
Grapefruit & Melon	Herring	Squash		
Berries (all kinds)				
Peaches (with skin)				

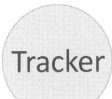
PRE-NATAL *Visits*

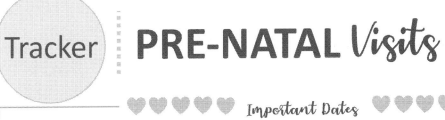

Important Dates

Keep track of your pre-natal appointments and include a summary of each visit.

		Summary of Appointment
Date		
How far along?		
Your Weight		
Blood Pressure		
Fetal Heart Rate		
Doctor		

NOTES:

Next Appointment.:

		Summary of Appointment
Date		
How far along?		
Your Weight		
Blood Pressure		
Fetal Heart Rate		
Doctor		

NOTES:

Next Appointment.:

		Summary of Appointment
Date		
How far along?		
Your Weight		
Blood Pressure		
Fetal Heart Rate		
Doctor		

NOTES:

Next Appointment.:

1-13 Weeks

FIRST *Trimester*

Journal your thoughts and feelings during each trimester so you can later reflect on your pregnancy journey.

HOW I FELT DURING MY FIRST TRIMESTER

MY FAVORITE MEMORIES

SYMPTOMS & CRAVINGS

ENERGY

SLEEP

CRAVINGS

MOODS

TO DO LIST: 1st TRIMESTER

FIRST TRIMESTER *Photos*

MEMORIES ARE FOREVER

14-27 Weeks

SECOND *Trimester*

HOW I FELT DURING MY SECOND TRIMESTER

MY FAVORITE MEMORIES

SYMPTOMS & CRAVINGS

ENERGY

SLEEP

CRAVINGS

MOODS

TO DO LIST: 2nd TRIMESTER

SECOND TRIMESTER *Photos*

MEMORIES ARE FOREVER

28-40 Weeks

THIRD Trimester

HOW I FELT DURING MY THIRD TRIMESTER

MY FAVORITE MEMORIES

SYMPTOMS & CRAVINGS

ENERGY

♥ ♥ ♥ ♥ ♥ ♥

SLEEP

♥ ♥ ♥ ♥ ♥ ♥

CRAVINGS

♥ ♥ ♥ ♥ ♥ ♥

MOODS

♥ ♥ ♥ ♥ ♥ ♥

TO DO LIST: 3rd TRIMESTER

THIRD TRIMESTER *Photos*

MEMORIES ARE FOREVER

MY BABY *Shower*

BABY SHOWER PHOTOS

GAMES PLAYED

ON THE MENU

HIGHLIGHTS & MEMORIES

MY BABY *Shower Gifts*

Keep track of your baby shower gifts and send thank you notes

NAME	GIFT	ADDRESS	SENT?
			☐
			☐
			☐
			☐
			☐
			☐
			☐
			☐
			☐
			☐
			☐
			☐
			☐
			☐
			☐
			☐

NURSERY *Planner*

♥ ♥

COLOR SCHEME IDEAS:

ITEM TO PURCHASE	PRICE	NOTES

FURNITURE IDEAS

DECORATIVE IDEAS

BABY NAME *Ideas*

TOP 3 BOY NAMES			

NAME MEANINGS

TOP 3 GIRL NAMES			

NAME MEANINGS

BABY NAME RESOURCES (LIST YOUR FAVORITE PARENTING & PREGNANCY WEBSITES):		

OTHER BOY NAME POSSIBILITIES	OTHER GIRL NAME POSSIBILITES

HOSPITAL *Checklist*

FOR ME	FOR PARTNER	FOR BABY

PREGNANCY SHOPPING *List*

BABY CLOTHING

SUPPLIES/MEDICATION

FURNITURE/TOYS

FIRST TRIMESTER SHOPPING

SECOND TRIMESTER SHOPPING

THIRD TRIMESTER SHOPPING

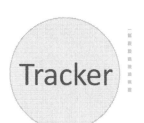

Tracker

FETAL *Movement*

Starting around week 16, keep track of when you feel your baby move.

WEEK 16	TIME	NOTES
MON		
TUE		
WED		
THU		
FRI		
SAT		
SUN		

WEEK 17	TIME	NOTES
MON		
TUE		
WED		
THU		
FRI		
SAT		
SUN		

WEEK 18	TIME	NOTES
MON		
TUE		
WED		
THU		
FRI		
SAT		
SUN		

WEEK 19	TIME	NOTES
MON		
TUE		
WED		
THU		
FRI		
SAT		
SUN		

WEEK 20	TIME	NOTES
MON		
TUE		
WED		
THU		
FRI		
SAT		
SUN		

WEEK 21	TIME	NOTES
MON		
TUE		
WED		
THU		
FRI		
SAT		
SUN		

WEEK 22	TIME	NOTES
MON		
TUE		
WED		
THU		
FRI		
SAT		
SUN		

WEEK 23	TIME	NOTES
MON		
TUE		
WED		
THU		
FRI		
SAT		
SUN		

WEEK 24	TIME	NOTES
MON		
TUE		
WED		
THU		
FRI		
SAT		
SUN		

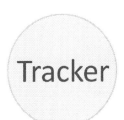

Tracker

FETAL Movement

♥ ♥ ♥ ♥ ♥ ♥ ♥ ♥ ♥ ♥ ♥ ♥ ♥ ♥ ♥ ♥ ♥ ♥ ♥ ♥

WEEK 25	TIME	NOTES
MON		
TUE		
WED		
THU		
FRI		
SAT		
SUN		

WEEK 26	TIME	NOTES
MON		
TUE		
WED		
THU		
FRI		
SAT		
SUN		

WEEK 27	TIME	NOTES
MON		
TUE		
WED		
THU		
FRI		
SAT		
SUN		

WEEK 28	TIME	NOTES
MON		
TUE		
WED		
THU		
FRI		
SAT		
SUN		

WEEK 29	TIME	NOTES
MON		
TUE		
WED		
THU		
FRI		
SAT		
SUN		

WEEK 30	TIME	NOTES
MON		
TUE		
WED		
THU		
FRI		
SAT		
SUN		

WEEK 31	TIME	NOTES
MON		
TUE		
WED		
THU		
FRI		
SAT		
SUN		

WEEK 32	TIME	NOTES
MON		
TUE		
WED		
THU		
FRI		
SAT		
SUN		

WEEK 33	TIME	NOTES
MON		
TUE		
WED		
THU		
FRI		
SAT		
SUN		

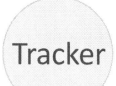

Tracker

FETAL *Movement*

WEEK 34	TIME	NOTES
MON		
TUE		
WED		
THU		
FRI		
SAT		
SUN		

WEEK 35	TIME	NOTES
MON		
TUE		
WED		
THU		
FRI		
SAT		
SUN		

WEEK 36	TIME	NOTES
MON		
TUE		
WED		
THU		
FRI		
SAT		
SUN		

WEEK 37	TIME	NOTES
MON		
TUE		
WED		
THU		
FRI		
SAT		
SUN		

WEEK 38	TIME	NOTES
MON		
TUE		
WED		
THU		
FRI		
SAT		
SUN		

WEEK 39	TIME	NOTES
MON		
TUE		
WED		
THU		
FRI		
SAT		
SUN		

WEEK 40	TIME	NOTES
MON		
TUE		
WED		
THU		
FRI		
SAT		
SUN		

NOTES		

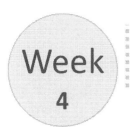

Week 4

PREGNANCY *Journal*

Your baby is the size of a poppy seed!

TOTAL WEIGHT GAIN

BELLY MEASUREMENT

BABY BUMP PHOTO

WEEKLY REFLECTIONS

SYMPTOMS & CRAVINGS

WHAT I WANT TO REMEMBER MOST

I'M MOST EXCITED ABOUT

I'M MOST NERVOUS ABOUT

Dear Baby,

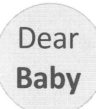

PREGNANCY *Journal*

TODAY'S DATE

WEEKS PREGNANT

HOW I'M FEELING TODAY

What I want you to know

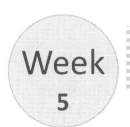
PREGNANCY *Journal*

Your baby is the size of a peppercorn!

TOTAL WEIGHT GAIN

5lbs

BELLY MEASUREMENT

BABY BUMP PHOTO

WEEKLY REFLECTIONS

In shock. I'm pregnant and never believed that I could. I honestly went from depression to acceptance. Once that happened, here comes baby!

SYMPTOMS & CRAVINGS

I'm very tired/sleepy. Not craving much.

WHAT I WANT TO REMEMBER MOST

how I felt when I saw the 2 lines on the pregnancy test. Also how Isaac reacted and the positive changes he's making

I'M MOST EXCITED ABOUT

my baby's health & heartbeat

I'M MOST NERVOUS ABOUT

the effect my fibroids will have

Dear Baby,

Wow! I can't believe you've made your way into my belly! Thank you for choosing me to be your mom. I promise to nurture you as you grow inside of me. I am your home.

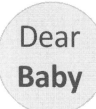

PREGNANCY *Journal*

TODAY'S DATE

WEEKS PREGNANT

HOW I'M FEELING TODAY

What I want you to know

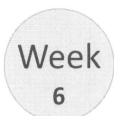

Week 6

PREGNANCY *Journal*

Your baby is the size of a sweet pea!

TOTAL WEIGHT GAIN
5 lbs

BELLY MEASUREMENT

BABY BUMP PHOTO

WEEKLY REFLECTIONS

This week I took it easy. I've been very exhausted. I didn't crack open not one book or assignment!

SYMPTOMS & CRAVINGS

Fatigue and not really any cravings

WHAT I WANT TO REMEMBER MOST

How stress free I remained. And how your dad + I did our best to provide.

I'M MOST EXCITED ABOUT

hearing your heartbeat

I'M MOST NERVOUS ABOUT

where we will live

Dear Baby,

I love you. You're growing and I'm so excited you've chosen me! Thank you.

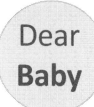

PREGNANCY *Journal*

Dear Baby

TODAY'S DATE

WEEKS PREGNANT

6

HOW I'M FEELING TODAY

tired + hungry

Week 6 I really took it easy. I didn't do much work and I also took a much needed break from school. I'm working hard to make sure we're good.

What I want you to know

You're sucking the energy out of me before you're physically here! I'm happy about it because all I get to do is eat and sleep. 2 things I love to do! I must stay active though. I can't be getting too big.

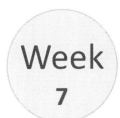

Week 7 · PREGNANCY *Journal*

Your baby is the size of a blueberry!

TOTAL WEIGHT GAIN

BELLY MEASUREMENT

BABY BUMP PHOTO

WEEKLY REFLECTIONS

Future life changes for me and Isaac. Working, going to school, and being pregnant is a lot. I am honestly wanting to keep to myself more. I am getting tired of everyones input. My pregnancy is specific to me.

SYMPTOMS & CRAVINGS

tired, beginning to feel emotional, just craving food

WHAT I WANT TO REMEMBER MOST

MOM + DAD HEARD YOUR HEARTBEAT TODAY!! Mommy SHED TEARS!

I'M MOST EXCITED ABOUT

seeing you develop! And discovering your sex (different from your gender)

I'M MOST NERVOUS ABOUT

Telling your Grandma. But very excited.

Dear Baby,

You got heart! Literally and metaphorically. I felt the presence of God when I heard your heart beating. You are strong and gentle. I Love you. Dad says he loves you too.

Dear Baby

PREGNANCY Journal

♥♥♥♥♥♥♥♥♥♥♥♥♥♥♥♥♥♥♥♥♥♥♥♥

TODAY'S DATE

11/9/21

WEEKS PREGNANT

7 wks 3 days

HOW I'M FEELING TODAY

Excited Blessed
Loved
Chosen

Today I got to see you and hear your heart beat! Wow! I am so grateful to God that my womb has been chosen as your home. I cried when I heard that strong little heart of yours. I recorded our encounter so that your daddy could see and hear you too! Because of the Pandemic, he's not allowed to come into the room to see you. I still made sure to document the experience so that he can feel the joy I felt. I'm so blessed. I'm very grateful. I will continue to make sure my womb, your home, is as comfortable and healthy as possible. Mommy does have a small fibroid and a small ovarian cyst. (L) There's nothing to worry about though because everything will be just fine.

♥♥♥♥♥♥♥♥♥♥♥♥♥♥♥♥♥♥♥♥♥♥

What I want you to know

I want you to know that against all odds, you can persevere and triumph over any and all obstacles! Remember to be strong and gentle. That's very important. It is beneficial to be soft and hard. Believe that keeping God in your mind, heart, and soul will allow you to achieve all your goals.
Asé! pronounced A-shay!

I Love You. We Love You.

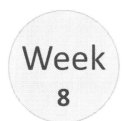

Week 8

PREGNANCY *Journal*

Your baby is the size of a raspberry!

TOTAL WEIGHT GAIN	BELLY MEASUREMENT

WEEKLY REFLECTIONS

I really need to take time for myself! I'm doing a lot and I need to relax. I'm also not wanting to talk to talk to people like that.

SYMPTOMS & CRAVINGS

Exhaustion

BABY BUMP PHOTO

WHAT I WANT TO REMEMBER MOST

I want to remember the peaceful times! I want to remember the quiet moments to myself.

I'M MOST EXCITED ABOUT

Seeing my baby's arms, legs, and head develop!

I'M MOST NERVOUS ABOUT

Stress! And not relaxing

Dear Baby,

Mama needs to set boundaries! For me, for you, and for Daddy. I want to enjoy each moment we have together.

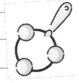

Dear Baby

PREGNANCY Journal

TODAY'S DATE

11/17/21

WEEKS PREGNANT

8 weeks 4 days

HOW I'M FEELING TODAY

Exhausted Sick
Lazy Itchy
Irritated restless

I'm doing too much and not enough at the same time. Too much of things that are not a priority which leaves me with no energy for the stuff I'm supposed to be doing. I guess it just always feels like it's something to do. I need to rest so that I have energy to give you. My eczema has been acting up bad, due to lack of rest and changes in eating. I am just falling off and I don't like that I'm getting back on. Which means more attention to myself and my baby, and less attention to others.

What I want you to know

I will protect you at any and all costs! No one and nothing takes priority over you. Your daddy and you are my #1 priorities and I will do all that I can to make sure boundaries are set for our family and that they're also respected! Anyone outside of the Bulbulia household takes a backseat! I got you baby! Now + forever.

And always remember that you are guided by your ancestors. They also protect you and us.

Asé.

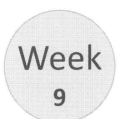

Week 9 · PREGNANCY Journal

Your baby is the size of a grape!

TOTAL WEIGHT GAIN: 2lbs 162lbs

BELLY MEASUREMENT:

BABY BUMP PHOTO

WEEKLY REFLECTIONS

We had our first Thanksgiving on Nov. 25, 2021! I don't like to call it thanksgiving since its historical context is about white men slaughtering Native Americans. But the meaning of it for our family is to gather, give thanks and be grateful! Also, to eat good!

SYMPTOMS & CRAVINGS

A tiny bit of nausea and extreme fatigue (or laziness) lowkey breathing heavier when I do certain things

WHAT I WANT TO REMEMBER MOST

The love and attention I gave to you in my womb.

I'M MOST EXCITED ABOUT

finally discovering your gender

I'M MOST NERVOUS ABOUT

birth defects. Although your dad and I will love you no matter what.

Dear Baby,

You're making Mommy's tummy bigger and I love it! Although I'm still a bit self-conscious, every roll is worth knowing you're here and you're healthy.

I love you ♡

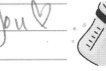

PREGNANCY *Journal*

♥♥♥♥♥♥♥♥♥♥♥♥♥♥♥♥♥♥♥♥♥♥♥♥

TODAY'S DATE

11/29/21

WEEKS PREGNANT

9 weeks

HOW I'M FEELING TODAY

mentally drained

I am mentally exausted! Over the past month, I have severely neglected my studies, and mildly neglect my work and household. I'm just having to give so much mental capacity elsewhere, my brain feels like its going to explode! The semester is almost over and I couldn't be happier! I know this will all be worth it in a couple of years, but dang its tiring right now! ><

♥♥♥♥♥♥♥♥♥♥♥♥♥♥♥♥♥♥♥♥♥♥♥♥

What I want you to know

Never give up! You can take a break and come back to it, but never give up on what it takes to achieve your goals. No matter how hard it is, remember that it could always be worse. Be grateful for the journey, and remember to feel your emotions. You are a spiritual being living a human experience. Having feelings is a part of who you are. Make sure to Nurture your emotions and others will also.

Week 10

PREGNANCY *Journal*

Your baby is the size of a prune!

TOTAL WEIGHT GAIN

BELLY MEASUREMENT

BABY BUMP PHOTO

WEEKLY REFLECTIONS

Close to the end of school!

SYMPTOMS & CRAVINGS

Pineapple and pizza

WHAT I WANT TO REMEMBER MOST

Seeing my belly bump grow.

I'M MOST EXCITED ABOUT

The next ultrasound

I'M MOST NERVOUS ABOUT

Getting through the first trimester

Dear Baby,

Time sure is going by fast! Already over 2 months into the pregnancy. I hope you can feel the love my dad and I are showing you. I hope you can feel it. We love you so much.

Dear Baby

PREGNANCY *Journal*

♥ ♥

TODAY'S DATE

WEEKS PREGNANT

HOW I'M FEELING TODAY

Overwhelmed

Feeling a bit stressed as finals are approaching. I have little to no energy to complete any tasks. I'm hoping to get back to my energized self and taking better care of my body.

What I want you to know

I'm doing all that I can to keep a balanced life. It is hard though. Work, school, you, your dad. I don't feel like myself somedays and that is okay. I know that it's temporary. I love you and your dad. Mom is just feeling overwhelmed.

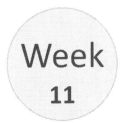

Week 11

PREGNANCY *Journal*

Your baby is the size of a lime!

TOTAL WEIGHT GAIN

BELLY MEASUREMENT

BABY BUMP PHOTO

WEEKLY REFLECTIONS

Finals week! I'm done with my first semester of grad school. Very proud of myself.

SYMPTOMS & CRAVINGS

Pizza, Fatigue

WHAT I WANT TO REMEMBER MOST

The effort I put into school

I'M MOST EXCITED ABOUT

Getting my grades back

I'M MOST NERVOUS ABOUT

Not passing all classes with A's and B's

Dear Baby,

Always remember to try your best! No matter what life throws at you, you have the strength and intelligence to persevere. And always remember that your family and ancestors got your back!

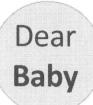

PREGNANCY *Journal*

TODAY'S DATE

WEEKS PREGNANT

11 weeks

HOW I'M FEELING TODAY

relieved

I'm happy that I've finished my first semester of grad school. So much happened this semester. Good and sad.
All in all, I'm always grateful for the good and not so good things that happen. Because everything happens for a reason.

What I want you to know

University isn't for everyone! But education will take you very far, to places you can imagine.
Even if you don't decide to go to a University as long as you obtain a skill, whether that's a certificate or an AA degree, always strive for the best and to advance in your career.

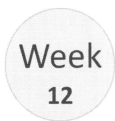

Week 12

PREGNANCY *Journal*

Your baby is the size of a plum!

TOTAL WEIGHT GAIN

BELLY MEASUREMENT

BABY BUMP PHOTO

WEEKLY REFLECTIONS

SYMPTOMS & CRAVINGS

WHAT I WANT TO REMEMBER MOST

I'M MOST EXCITED ABOUT

I'M MOST NERVOUS ABOUT

Dear Baby,

12 WEEKS

ULTRASOUND *Scan*

ULTRASOUND PHOTO

ULTRASOUND RESULTS

BABY'S LENGTH:

BABY'S WEIGHT:

BPD:

DUE DATE:

Notes

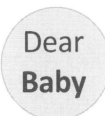

PREGNANCY *Journal*

TODAY'S DATE

WEEKS PREGNANT

HOW I'M FEELING TODAY

What I want you to know

Week 13

PREGNANCY *Journal*

Your baby is the size of a peach!

TOTAL WEIGHT GAIN

BELLY MEASUREMENT

BABY BUMP PHOTO

WEEKLY REFLECTIONS

SYMPTOMS & CRAVINGS

WHAT I WANT TO REMEMBER MOST

I'M MOST EXCITED ABOUT

I'M MOST NERVOUS ABOUT

Dear Baby,

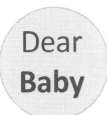

PREGNANCY *Journal*

♥♥♥♥♥♥♥♥♥♥♥♥♥♥♥♥♥♥♥♥♥♥♥♥

TODAY'S DATE

WEEKS PREGNANT

HOW I'M FEELING TODAY

What I want you to know

Week 14 | PREGNANCY Journal

Your baby is the size of a lemon!

TOTAL WEIGHT GAIN

BELLY MEASUREMENT

BABY BUMP PHOTO

WEEKLY REFLECTIONS

Insecure about motherhood and the future
Scared about Baby's health
Worried about what's to come
Trying not to stres
Feeling lazy
Catching Covid-19

SYMPTOMS & CRAVINGS

extremely tired and feeling hot

WHAT I WANT TO REMEMBER MOST

I want to remember the good times between your Dad and I

I'M MOST EXCITED ABOUT

Seeing your face

I'M MOST NERVOUS ABOUT

Keeping you healthy in the womb

Dear Baby,

Mom is trying her best to stay healthy and to remain stress-free. I want you to enjoy your time in my womb. I can't control anything but what I do and how I respond to things. Always remember that for you too.

TODAY'S DATE

1/1/2022

WEEKS PREGNANT

14

HOW I'M FEELING TODAY

Worried but calmer than usual

Happy New Year! We're officially in the year 2022. The year you will make your grand entrance into the physical world. But I've been worried lately. I've been spotting (little amounts of blood coming from inside my vagina), and that had me scared. The doctor said that you're okay as long as it's not a lot of blood. I've been put on bed rest the past week. I love you so much baby and I want to do all that I can to make sure you're developing properly. I know that I can do more and I will. I also had a cold. I think your dad passed it onto me. As of today I feel completely better. I do need to take proper precautions though.

What I want you to know

Your Dad and I love each other. That's what it took for you to get here. We love you even more. No matter what Dad and Mom go through, you will always be the light in our lives; the love in our hearts. Always and forever my baby. ♡

Week 15

PREGNANCY *Journal*

Your baby is the size of an apple!

TOTAL WEIGHT GAIN

BELLY MEASUREMENT

BABY BUMP PHOTO

WEEKLY REFLECTIONS

SYMPTOMS & CRAVINGS

WHAT I WANT TO REMEMBER MOST

I'M MOST EXCITED ABOUT

I'M MOST NERVOUS ABOUT

Dear Baby,

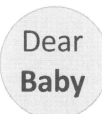

Dear Baby

PREGNANCY *Journal*

TODAY'S DATE

WEEKS PREGNANT

HOW I'M FEELING TODAY

What I want you to know

Week 16

PREGNANCY *Journal*

Your baby is the size of an avocado!

TOTAL WEIGHT GAIN

BELLY MEASUREMENT

BABY BUMP PHOTO

WEEKLY REFLECTIONS

SYMPTOMS & CRAVINGS

WHAT I WANT TO REMEMBER MOST

I'M MOST EXCITED ABOUT

I'M MOST NERVOUS ABOUT

Dear Baby,

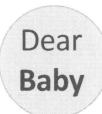

PREGNANCY *Journal*

TODAY'S DATE

WEEKS PREGNANT

HOW I'M FEELING TODAY

What I want you to know

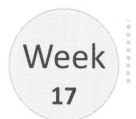

Week 17

PREGNANCY *Journal*

Your baby is the size of a pear!

TOTAL WEIGHT GAIN

BELLY MEASUREMENT

BABY BUMP PHOTO

WEEKLY REFLECTIONS

SYMPTOMS & CRAVINGS

WHAT I WANT TO REMEMBER MOST

I'M MOST EXCITED ABOUT

I'M MOST NERVOUS ABOUT

Dear Baby,

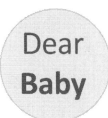

PREGNANCY *Journal*

TODAY'S DATE

WEEKS PREGNANT

HOW I'M FEELING TODAY

What I want you to know

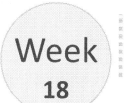

Week 18

PREGNANCY *Journal*

Your baby is the size of a sweet potato!

TOTAL WEIGHT GAIN	BELLY MEASUREMENT

BABY BUMP PHOTO

WEEKLY REFLECTIONS

SYMPTOMS & CRAVINGS

WHAT I WANT TO REMEMBER MOST

I'M MOST EXCITED ABOUT

I'M MOST NERVOUS ABOUT

Dear Baby,

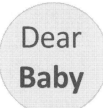

PREGNANCY *Journal*

♥♥♥♥♥♥♥♥♥♥♥♥♥♥♥♥♥♥♥♥♥♥♥♥

**TODAY'S
DATE**

**WEEKS
PREGNANT**

**HOW I'M
FEELING TODAY**

♥♥♥♥♥♥♥♥♥♥♥♥♥♥♥♥♥♥♥♥♥♥♥♥♥♥♥♥♥♥♥♥

What I want you to know

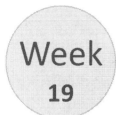

Week 19

PREGNANCY *Journal*

Your baby is the size of a mango!

TOTAL WEIGHT GAIN

BELLY MEASUREMENT

BABY BUMP PHOTO

WEEKLY REFLECTIONS

SYMPTOMS & CRAVINGS

WHAT I WANT TO REMEMBER MOST

I'M MOST EXCITED ABOUT

I'M MOST NERVOUS ABOUT

Dear Baby,

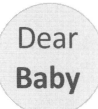

PREGNANCY *Journal*

TODAY'S DATE

WEEKS PREGNANT

HOW I'M FEELING TODAY

What I want you to know

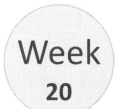

Week 20

PREGNANCY *Journal*

Your baby is the size of a banana!

TOTAL WEIGHT GAIN

BELLY MEASUREMENT

BABY BUMP PHOTO

WEEKLY REFLECTIONS

SYMPTOMS & CRAVINGS

WHAT I WANT TO REMEMBER MOST

I'M MOST EXCITED ABOUT

I'M MOST NERVOUS ABOUT

Dear Baby,

20 WEEKS

ULTRASOUND *Scan*

♥♥♥♥♥♥♥♥♥♥♥♥♥♥♥♥♥♥♥♥♥♥

ULTRASOUND PHOTO

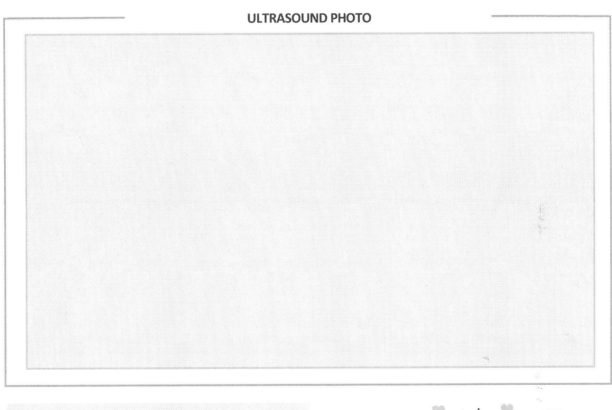

ULTRASOUND RESULTS

BABY'S LENGTH:

BABY'S WEIGHT:

BPD:

DUE DATE:

♥ *Notes* ♥

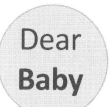

Dear Baby

PREGNANCY *Journal*

TODAY'S DATE

WEEKS PREGNANT
20 + 6

HOW I'M FEELING TODAY
Pretty and great

Hey baby! I know its been a while since I've written about you in the journal. So many ups and downs have happened over the past few weeks. You have Mommy feeling so emotional. It's okay though. I need to feel all the feelings. And remember that it's good and necessary for you to feel your feelings as well. Don't ever let anyone else tell you otherwise. You are a human and you have feelings. You will feel emotions. And you are entitled to each and every one of them. When you're older, and start dating, you make sure to be with someone that nurtures those feelings. Your Mom and Dad always will.

What I want you to know

Your Mom + Dad loves you unconditionally. We will always do our best to be emotionally present. You can confide in us about anything without judgement. We promise to nurture your feelings. Your emotional development is important to us. We love you so much Baby. ♡

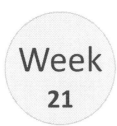

Week 21

PREGNANCY *Journal*

Your baby is the size of a carrot!

TOTAL WEIGHT GAIN

BELLY MEASUREMENT

BABY BUMP PHOTO

WEEKLY REFLECTIONS

SYMPTOMS & CRAVINGS

WHAT I WANT TO REMEMBER MOST

I'M MOST EXCITED ABOUT

I'M MOST NERVOUS ABOUT

Dear Baby,

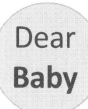

Dear Baby

PREGNANCY *Journal*

TODAY'S DATE

WEEKS PREGNANT

HOW I'M FEELING TODAY

What I want you to know

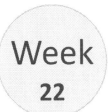

Week 22

PREGNANCY *Journal*

Your baby is the size of a papaya!

TOTAL WEIGHT GAIN

BELLY MEASUREMENT

BABY BUMP PHOTO

WEEKLY REFLECTIONS

SYMPTOMS & CRAVINGS

WHAT I WANT TO REMEMBER MOST

I'M MOST EXCITED ABOUT

I'M MOST NERVOUS ABOUT

Dear Baby,

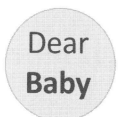

PREGNANCY *Journal*

TODAY'S DATE

WEEKS PREGNANT

HOW I'M FEELING TODAY

What I want you to know

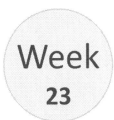

Week 23

PREGNANCY *Journal*

Your baby is the size of a grapefruit!

TOTAL WEIGHT GAIN

BELLY MEASUREMENT

BABY BUMP PHOTO

WEEKLY REFLECTIONS

SYMPTOMS & CRAVINGS

WHAT I WANT TO REMEMBER MOST

I'M MOST EXCITED ABOUT

I'M MOST NERVOUS ABOUT

Dear Baby,

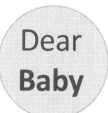

Dear Baby

PREGNANCY *Journal*

TODAY'S DATE

WEEKS PREGNANT

HOW I'M FEELING TODAY

What I want you to know

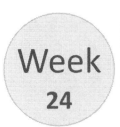

Week 24

PREGNANCY *Journal*

Your baby is the size of a cantaloupe!

TOTAL WEIGHT GAIN

BELLY MEASUREMENT

BABY BUMP PHOTO

WEEKLY REFLECTIONS

SYMPTOMS & CRAVINGS

WHAT I WANT TO REMEMBER MOST

I'M MOST EXCITED ABOUT

I'M MOST NERVOUS ABOUT

Dear Baby,

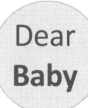

Dear Baby

PREGNANCY *Journal*

TODAY'S DATE

WEEKS PREGNANT

HOW I'M FEELING TODAY

What I want you to know

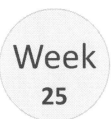

Week 25

PREGNANCY *Journal*

Your baby is the size of a cauliflower!

TOTAL WEIGHT GAIN

BELLY MEASUREMENT

BABY BUMP PHOTO

WEEKLY REFLECTIONS

SYMPTOMS & CRAVINGS

WHAT I WANT TO REMEMBER MOST

I'M MOST EXCITED ABOUT

I'M MOST NERVOUS ABOUT

Dear Baby,

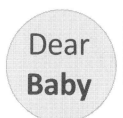

Dear **Baby**

PREGNANCY *Journal*

TODAY'S DATE

WEEKS PREGNANT

HOW I'M FEELING TODAY

What I want you to know

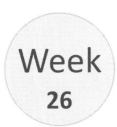

Week 26

PREGNANCY *Journal*

Your baby is the size of a head of lettuce!

TOTAL WEIGHT GAIN

BELLY MEASUREMENT

BABY BUMP PHOTO

WEEKLY REFLECTIONS

SYMPTOMS & CRAVINGS

WHAT I WANT TO REMEMBER MOST

I'M MOST EXCITED ABOUT

I'M MOST NERVOUS ABOUT

Dear Baby,

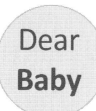

Dear Baby

PREGNANCY *Journal*

♥♥♥♥♥♥♥♥♥♥♥♥♥♥♥♥♥♥

TODAY'S DATE

WEEKS PREGNANT

HOW I'M FEELING TODAY

What I want you to know

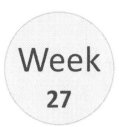

Week 27

PREGNANCY *Journal*

Your baby is the size of a rutabaga!

TOTAL WEIGHT GAIN

BELLY MEASUREMENT

BABY BUMP PHOTO

WEEKLY REFLECTIONS

SYMPTOMS & CRAVINGS

WHAT I WANT TO REMEMBER MOST

I'M MOST EXCITED ABOUT

I'M MOST NERVOUS ABOUT

Dear Baby,

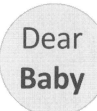

PREGNANCY *Journal*

TODAY'S DATE

WEEKS PREGNANT

HOW I'M FEELING TODAY

What I want you to know

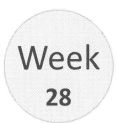

Week 28

PREGNANCY *Journal*

Your baby is the size of an eggplant!

**TOTAL
WEIGHT GAIN**

**BELLY
MEASUREMENT**

BABY BUMP PHOTO

WEEKLY REFLECTIONS

SYMPTOMS & CRAVINGS

WHAT I WANT TO REMEMBER MOST

I'M MOST EXCITED ABOUT

I'M MOST NERVOUS ABOUT

Dear Baby,

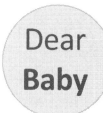

Dear Baby

PREGNANCY *Journal*

♥ ♥ ♥ ♥ ♥ ♥ ♥ ♥ ♥ ♥ ♥ ♥ ♥ ♥ ♥ ♥ ♥ ♥ ♥

TODAY'S DATE

WEEKS PREGNANT

HOW I'M FEELING TODAY

♥ ♥

What I want you to know

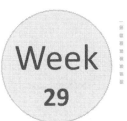

Week 29

PREGNANCY *Journal*

Your baby is the size of an acorn squash!

TOTAL WEIGHT GAIN

BELLY MEASUREMENT

BABY BUMP PHOTO

WEEKLY REFLECTIONS

SYMPTOMS & CRAVINGS

WHAT I WANT TO REMEMBER MOST

I'M MOST EXCITED ABOUT

I'M MOST NERVOUS ABOUT

Dear Baby,

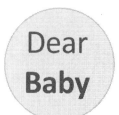

Dear Baby

PREGNANCY *Journal*

♥ ♥ ♥ ♥ ♥ ♥ ♥ ♥ ♥ ♥ ♥ ♥ ♥ ♥ ♥ ♥ ♥ ♥

TODAY'S DATE

WEEKS PREGNANT

HOW I'M FEELING TODAY

What I want you to know

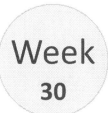

Week 30

PREGNANCY *Journal*

Your baby is the size of a cucumber!

TOTAL WEIGHT GAIN

BELLY MEASUREMENT

BABY BUMP PHOTO

WEEKLY REFLECTIONS

SYMPTOMS & CRAVINGS

WHAT I WANT TO REMEMBER MOST

I'M MOST EXCITED ABOUT

I'M MOST NERVOUS ABOUT

Dear Baby,

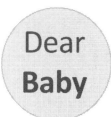

PREGNANCY *Journal*

TODAY'S DATE

WEEKS PREGNANT

HOW I'M FEELING TODAY

What I want you to know

Week 31

PREGNANCY *Journal*

Your baby is the size of a pineapple!

TOTAL WEIGHT GAIN

BELLY MEASUREMENT

BABY BUMP PHOTO

WEEKLY REFLECTIONS

SYMPTOMS & CRAVINGS

WHAT I WANT TO REMEMBER MOST

I'M MOST EXCITED ABOUT

I'M MOST NERVOUS ABOUT

Dear Baby,

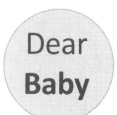

PREGNANCY *Journal*

TODAY'S DATE

WEEKS PREGNANT

HOW I'M FEELING TODAY

What I want you to know

PREGNANCY *Journal*

Your baby is the size of a squash!

TOTAL WEIGHT GAIN

BELLY MEASUREMENT

BABY BUMP PHOTO

WEEKLY REFLECTIONS

SYMPTOMS & CRAVINGS

WHAT I WANT TO REMEMBER MOST

I'M MOST EXCITED ABOUT

I'M MOST NERVOUS ABOUT

Dear Baby,

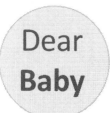

Dear Baby

PREGNANCY *Journal*

TODAY'S DATE

WEEKS PREGNANT

HOW I'M FEELING TODAY

What I want you to know

Week 33

PREGNANCY *Journal*

Your baby is the size of a durian!

TOTAL WEIGHT GAIN

BELLY MEASUREMENT

BABY BUMP PHOTO

WEEKLY REFLECTIONS

SYMPTOMS & CRAVINGS

WHAT I WANT TO REMEMBER MOST

I'M MOST EXCITED ABOUT

I'M MOST NERVOUS ABOUT

Dear Baby,

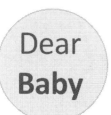

Dear Baby

PREGNANCY *Journal*

♥ ♥ ♥ ♥ ♥ ♥ ♥ ♥ ♥ ♥ ♥ ♥ ♥ ♥ ♥ ♥ ♥ ♥ ♥

TODAY'S DATE

WEEKS PREGNANT

HOW I'M FEELING TODAY

What I want you to know

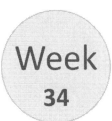

Week 34

PREGNANCY *Journal*

Your baby is the size of a butternut squash!

TOTAL WEIGHT GAIN

BELLY MEASUREMENT

BABY BUMP PHOTO

WEEKLY REFLECTIONS

SYMPTOMS & CRAVINGS

WHAT I WANT TO REMEMBER MOST

I'M MOST EXCITED ABOUT

I'M MOST NERVOUS ABOUT

Dear Baby,

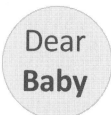

PREGNANCY *Journal*

TODAY'S DATE

WEEKS PREGNANT

HOW I'M FEELING TODAY

What I want you to know

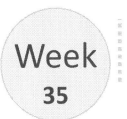

Week 35

PREGNANCY *Journal*

Your baby is the size of a coconut!

TOTAL WEIGHT GAIN

BELLY MEASUREMENT

BABY BUMP PHOTO

WEEKLY REFLECTIONS

SYMPTOMS & CRAVINGS

WHAT I WANT TO REMEMBER MOST

I'M MOST EXCITED ABOUT

I'M MOST NERVOUS ABOUT

Dear Baby,

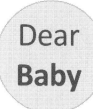

Dear Baby

PREGNANCY *Journal*

♥♥♥♥♥♥♥♥♥♥♥♥♥♥♥♥♥♥♥♥♥

TODAY'S DATE

WEEKS PREGNANT

HOW I'M FEELING TODAY

What I want you to know

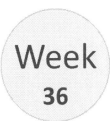

Week 36

PREGNANCY *Journal*

Your baby is the size of a honeydew melon!

TOTAL WEIGHT GAIN

BELLY MEASUREMENT

BABY BUMP PHOTO

WEEKLY REFLECTIONS

SYMPTOMS & CRAVINGS

WHAT I WANT TO REMEMBER MOST

I'M MOST EXCITED ABOUT

I'M MOST NERVOUS ABOUT

Dear Baby,

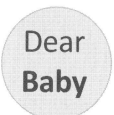

Dear Baby

PREGNANCY *Journal*

♥♥♥♥♥♥♥♥♥♥♥♥♥♥♥♥♥♥♥♥♥

TODAY'S DATE

WEEKS PREGNANT

HOW I'M FEELING TODAY

What I want you to know

PREGNANCY *Journal*

Your baby is the size of a Winter Melon!

TOTAL WEIGHT GAIN

BELLY MEASUREMENT

BABY BUMP PHOTO

WEEKLY REFLECTIONS

SYMPTOMS & CRAVINGS

WHAT I WANT TO REMEMBER MOST

I'M MOST EXCITED ABOUT

I'M MOST NERVOUS ABOUT

Dear Baby,

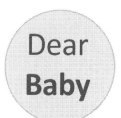

PREGNANCY *Journal*

TODAY'S DATE

WEEKS PREGNANT

HOW I'M FEELING TODAY

What I want you to know

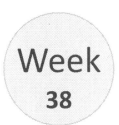

Week 38

PREGNANCY Journal

Your baby is the size of a pumpkin!

TOTAL WEIGHT GAIN

BELLY MEASUREMENT

BABY BUMP PHOTO

WEEKLY REFLECTIONS

SYMPTOMS & CRAVINGS

WHAT I WANT TO REMEMBER MOST

I'M MOST EXCITED ABOUT

I'M MOST NERVOUS ABOUT

Dear Baby,

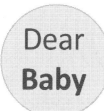

PREGNANCY *Journal*

TODAY'S DATE

WEEKS PREGNANT

HOW I'M FEELING TODAY

What I want you to know

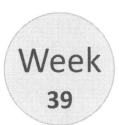

Week 39

PREGNANCY *Journal*

Your baby is the size of a watermelon!

TOTAL WEIGHT GAIN

BELLY MEASUREMENT

BABY BUMP PHOTO

WEEKLY REFLECTIONS

SYMPTOMS & CRAVINGS

WHAT I WANT TO REMEMBER MOST

I'M MOST EXCITED ABOUT

I'M MOST NERVOUS ABOUT

Dear Baby,

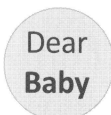

Dear Baby

PREGNANCY *Journal*

♥ ♥ ♥ ♥ ♥ ♥ ♥ ♥ ♥ ♥ ♥ ♥ ♥ ♥ ♥ ♥ ♥ ♥

TODAY'S DATE

WEEKS PREGNANT

HOW I'M FEELING TODAY

What I want you to know

PREGNANCY *Journal*

Your baby is the size of a jack fruit!

TOTAL WEIGHT GAIN

BELLY MEASUREMENT

BABY BUMP PHOTO

WEEKLY REFLECTIONS

SYMPTOMS & CRAVINGS

WHAT I WANT TO REMEMBER MOST

I'M MOST EXCITED ABOUT

I'M MOST NERVOUS ABOUT

Dear Baby,

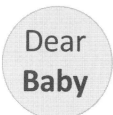

Dear Baby

PREGNANCY *Journal*

♥♥♥♥♥♥♥♥♥♥♥♥♥♥♥♥♥♥♥♥♥

**TODAY'S
DATE**

**WEEKS
PREGNANT**

**HOW I'M
FEELING TODAY**

What I want you to know

Made in the USA
Columbia, SC
28 October 2021